Griddle Low Carb:

20 Amazing Low Calorie Recipes

Table of Content

.

Introduction

Thank you for buying this book! The panini press griddler is a fantastic way to cook some of your favorites. It's quick, it's easy, and it's versatile. You should know that it's used for more than just making a delicious panini. However, when you buy one, you may think that you can only grill burgers and chicken on there. While those taste great, there's plenty of other recipes out there, and they'll make your mouth water. These treats are easy to make and are quite delicious! From breakfast, lunch, dinner, and dessert, this book will cover all meals, with five recipes for each of them.

Note that you don't necessarily have to have a Panini Press to cook these. Any indoor grill will work. For best results, however, a Panini Press is recommended. If you have a Foreman, it'll work too.

Chapter 1 – The Grilling Revolution

A long time ago, it used to be quite cumbersome to grill something. You had to set up a bulky grill, grab the coal, and light a fire. If weather conditions weren't ideal, there was no grilling for you. Indoor grills did exist, but they were for fancy restaurants.

But those times have changed. While nothing beats a hamburger over a flame, indoor grilling comes close. Indoor grills are relatively inexpensive and allow anyone to cook delicious recipes in no time at all. There are many indoor grills out there. Some lock in all the flavor, and some drain the fat for a healthier meal. There are panini presses out there that will give you a great panini, a grilled sandwich that doesn't use sliced bread. Once you have an indoor grill, you practically never have to eat out again.

However, many people undervalue their grills. They think that you can make a few sandwiches or meats, and that's it. But that's not the case! You can make a good meal using your grill. In the next few chapters, you'll learn about just a few of the recipes that you can cook with your panini press. These recipes don't necessarily require that, but it is recommended. All grills are made different, so check to see if your grill's surface is adjustable, if it has heat settings, or if it has a drip tray.

A few other tips are as follows:

1. Always preheat the grill before you cook. This should be common sense, but many people forget that. You want to expose the food to the temperature that it needs to cook all the time when it's cooking, so if it's less, it may be overcooked.

2. All griddles aren't created equal. Some may give off different temperatures than others. Some grills only have one set temperature. Some use numbers instead of words. Because of this, make sure to check your food when it's in the range of the recommended minutes. It may need more time, or it may need less. Do not mess it up by overcooking or undercooking your meal.

3. Make sure to check to see if your griddle is nonstick or not. If it's not, you need to grease up your grills so it doesn't stick. Use some fat-free cooking spray for best results.

4. Make sure to check the thickness of what you're grilling. If it's too thick, it may take longer to cook. If one food is thicker than the other, the grill may close its lid on one and not the other, cooking them unequally. Measure beforehand so you don't face the consequences.

5. Always clean after every use. This means that you should invest in a scraper so you can scrape your grill beforehand. Empty your drip tray on occasion too. If your grills are removable, you can use your dishwasher or sink for easy cleaning. Don't put it in the water if the grill is attached, however. Water may damage your unit.

6. Adjust your grill accordingly. Some recipes may require your grill to be flat, others tilted. See if your grill is adjustable beforehand.

7. Finally, have fun with what you cook. Remember that cooking can be about experimentation as well. Because of this, you may want to try some of your own recipes. Feel free to modify the provided recipes as well, and adjust to your liking. If you're a vegetarian or vegan, substitute the meats and dairy products. If you don't like a food, such as onions, take it out or replace it with something you do like. This book is merely a way get you

started, and the recipes aren't the end-all, be all. Adjust the amount of ingredients to your liking, and experiment.

Chapter 2 – A Grilled Breakfast

Breakfast is the most important meal of the day, and everyone strives for a hearty meal that will help them break the fast. But not everyone has the time to cook a great meal every day. Some may fix something quick, or nothing at all. However, you need a good meal if you want to survive the world, and because of this, you should make sure you're getting enough food. Indoor grilling can help with that.

There are plenty of breakfast dishes you can fix with your panini press or indoor grill, and they'll give you diner-quality meals for cheap and in no time at all. These recipes are quick and easy to make.

Bacon

The traditional way of cooking bacon is through the pan. However, you can get the same crispy results through a panini press. No having to worry about grease popping, either.

What You Need

- Six slices of raw bacon

Directions

1. Preheat the press to around medium-high, installing the drip pan if it has one. If it can tilt, make sure to do that first.

2. Place the bacon slices in a neat fashion, making sure they don't overlap. You may need to trim the bacon if your press is small.

3. After that, simply close the lid and wait for about 10-14 minutes.

4. If you have a grill where you can change the upper plate's height, adjust so that it barely touches the top of the bacon, for best results. Depending on the thickness, it may take more time.

5. Remove the strips once cooked and enjoy!

Delicious Hashbrowns

What You Need

- 30 oz of shredded potatoes, frozen.
- 1/3 cup of olice oil
- 1 tsp salt. Adjust to taste.
- ½ tsp of paprika
- ¼ tsp of black pepper
- Feel free to add cheese, jalapeños, diced ham, or anything else to the mix as well.

Directions

1. Set your press to medium-high heat.

2. Combine all ingredients in a large bowl, tossing as you do in order to combine.

3. Once the press is heated, spoon your mix on your press and close the lid tightly.

4. Cook for 5-10 minutes, depending on how crispy you like your hashbrowns. Remove from the press and add more mixture.

Health Omelet

If you want something filling in under 400 calories, this omelet will do it. At just 350 calories, it packs quite a punch of flavor.

What You Need

- ¼ cup of egg product, i.e. Egg Beaters
- ¼ cup diced onion
- 1 diced jalapeno
- 1 tbsp diced Roma tomato
- 1 tbsp of reduced fat cheese, preferably Mexican
- 1 diced red potato, about the size of a golf ball

- 2 sausage links
- Salt and pepper for taste
- Any kind of tobasco sauce to taste, optional
- Cooking spray

Directions

1. Heat your press to high. Spray it with the cooking spray. Dice your potato in even slices. Then, dice onion, jalapeno, and tomato. Put everything aside.

2. Shake your egg substitute, and pour it into the measuring cup. Put tomato and half of the peppers in the cup and stir. Add tobasco sauce if you want, and add salt and pepper too. Set it aside.

3. Put sausage and potatoes on the grill for five minutes. Then, add peppers and onions to the mix. After that, add your egg mixture.

4. By now grill should be at operating temperature. Place diced potatoes and sausage links on grill. After about 5 minutes, add diced peppers and onions to potatoes; mix with diced potatoes. Add egg product mixture to grill. Once sausage is done (about 6 minutes or so,) take them out. About ten minutes, the potatoes should be done, along with the omelet. Add potatoes and links to the omelet and serve.

Waffle Panini

Enough said. Best of all, this recipe has just 470 calories.

What You Need

- 4 lightly toasted frozen waffles, preferably whole grain.
- 2 lightly beaten large eggs
- 2 tbsp of butter, divided.
- 2 slices of cheese, preferably cheddar
- 2 cooked turkey sausage patties

Direction

1. Melt one tbsp. of butter and spread it in your skillet over medium-low heat.

2. Add eggs and cook for about four minutes, not stirring. Lower heat and cook for four minutes, covered. Removing from the heat and cut in half, topping each side with cheese.

3. Put egg, cheese, and sausage on two waffles, and then top with two waffles. Put it in your press over medium heat and put one tbsp. butter in the grill.

4. Cook for four minutes, turning once until waffle is golden brown and the cheese is melted.

Breakfast Burrito

What You Need

- 1 seeded and diced jalapeno
- 1 minced garlic clove
- 1 tbsp of fresh lime juice
- ½ tsp of salt, adjust to taste
- 2 pitted, peeled, and halved large avocadoes
- 2 tbs of fresh chopped cilantro
- 3 tbsp of olive oil. Add more for brushing
- 1 seeded and diced red bell pepper
- 1 seeded and diced green bell pepper
- ¾ lb of Yukon Gold potatoes, boiled and tendered, then diced
- Black pepper to taste
- 6 bacon slices
- 12 eggs
- 6 flour tortillas
- 6 oz grated cheddar cheese
- Sour cream and salsa to serve

Directions

1. Combine jalapeno, garlic, lime juice, and salt in a small bowl. Crush with a fork until you have a coarse paste.

2. Mix in the avocados and cilantro and mash into a lumpy paste. Set your guacamole aside.

3. In a nonstick frying pan over medium heat, add 2 tbsp of olive oil. Put in the bell peppers and fry, stirring on occasion for about 8-10 minutes.

4. Put in the potatoes and cook until warmed, which should be about 3-5 minutes.

5. Add salt and pepper and keep them warm.

6. Preheat your press on the panini setting.

7. Put the bacon in the press and close your lid. Cook until crispy, which should be about 4 minutes.

8. Drain grease on paper towels, and wipe off your press.

9. In another bowl, beat eggs, salt, and pepper.

10. In a frying pan over medium-high, warm 1 tbsp of olive oil.

11. Add your eggs and stir occasionally. Do it for 2-3 minutes or until curds appear.

12. Put a spoonful of the eggs in the center of your tortilla, and top with bell peppers and one crumbled bacon slice, as well as an ounce of cheese.

13. Roll it into a burrito and brush the outside with olive oil.

14. Put two burritos in your press and close the lid.

15. Cook for about 2-3 minutes, or until crispy.

16. Repeat for the remaining burritos.

17. Serve with salsa, sour cream, and guacamole.

Chapter 3 – Time for Lunch!

Lunch is considered by many to be the middle meal of the day, a sort of appetizer until dinner. However, that doesn't mean that you have to settle for less. With your panini press, you can make many delicious dishes that can be whipped up in minutes. After all, this is a griddle known for making sandwiches, but there are so many foods you can cook in addition to that. So why settle for less? This chapter will cover all the lunch classics, from chicken, burgers, and even the classic grilled cheese. With that, here are the recipes.

Chicken

This simple grilled recipe is low in calories and fat, but high in protein and taste!

What You Need

- 2 boneless and skinless chicken breasts, about ½" in thickness
- 1 tbsp of olive oil
- ½ tsp salt
- ½ tsp of black pepper
- ½ tap of paprika
- ½ tsp of parsley flakes

Directions:

1. Preheat press for about five minutes using the high setting.

2. Coat both sides of your chicken breasts with olive oil.

3. Mix paprika, parsley, and salt on a plate, and cover both sides with chicken generously. Poke chicken with a fork a few times.

4. Put meat into heated grill and grill for about five minutes, closing the lid.

5. After that, rotate meat about ¼ of a turn and cook for a couple more minutes. Make sure there is no pink in the middle.

6. Serve.

Homemade Pizza

This rustic-looking pizza is great for a quick lunch. And you can cook it on your grill.

What You Need

- Olive oil, for brushing
- Aluminum foil
- 1 lb of fresh pizza dough
- Pesto sauce
- Cheese, pepperoni, and whatever toppings you want.

Directions

1. Set your press to high and make sure it's flat.

2. Brush olive oil on foil in a 6-inch circle. Or, just use cooking spray.

3. Divide dough into 6 servings. Stretch dough into a circle.

4. Do it as thin as possible for easy cooking.

5. Add your sauce to the pizzas.

6. Top with cheese and add whatever ingredients you want to it.

7. lace on pizza, and adjust the lid so it's barely hovering over the pizza.

8. Cook for about 6-8 minutes, and then serve.

Burgers

This recipe is a classic, and you can make great hamburgers using your panini press.

What You Need

- Ground Beef, around 80-85% lean
- Seasonings, to taste

Directions

1. Heat press on a medium high setting.

2. Season your beef with whatever you want, and then form into patties.

3. Make sure they have about the same size and thickness.

4. Put burgers on grill and close the lid.

5. Cook for about 6-8 minutes, and then add them to your buns.

6. Top with whatever you like.

7. Make sure to scrape the grill afterwards.

8. If you want to grill your buns, put them in for about a couple minutes.

Turkey Quesadilla

This recipe is cheesy and delicious! With your panini press, you can make it in no time at all too!

What You Need

- 1 flour tortilla
- 2 slices of deli turkey
- 1 handful of shredded cheese
- Add other ingredients to your liking, such as veggies if you wish.

Directions

1. Preheat on medium high, and while it's heating, sprinkle half of your cheese on one half of the tortilla.

2. Add turkey to the top of shredded cheese, and put the remaining cheese on top of your turkey.

3. Add any other ingredients that you wish.

4. Once that's done, fold your tortilla in half.

5. Put it in your press and close the lid.

6. Cook for about a minute, or until everything's melted. Take off the press and serve.

Basil-Lemon Grilled Cheese

A great twist on an old recipe, this will have everyone talking.

What You Need

- 1 cup of shredded mozzarella
- 2 oz of crumbled feta
- 2 tsp grated lemon zest
- 2 tsp chopped basil, fresh
- 1 tbsp of extra-virgin olive oil
- 8 slices of Italian bread (or sourdough,) sliced from a bakery load.

Directions

1. Heat your press to medium high.

2. While it's heating, toss your cheeses, lemon, and basil in a medium bowl.

3. Brush olive oil on two slices of your bread to give the outside some flavor.

4. Flip over a slice and top with cheese mix. Close the sandwich with your other bread slice, making sure the oiled size is up.

5. Grill two panini with the lid closed for about five minutes or until bread is toasted and cheese is melted.

Chapter 4 – Dinner Time!

Dinner is considered by many to be the big meal that restores your energy after a long day. Whether you're getting home from work or slaving over a stove all day, dinner is said to be the reward at the end of the tunnel.

As such, there are five great recipes here to make dinnertime more fun. Best of all, many of these recipes can be cooked in a flash. Because of this, you don't have to worry about wasting too much time over the stove, and instead do the things you like. Whether it's for your spouse, for your kids, or for yourself, you can make a satisfying meal using your indoor grill.

Grilled Shrimp

Seafood is great on the grill, and you can make grilled shrimp that is sure to please. You can serve this with a variety of dishes, so mix and match if you want.

What You Need

- 1 lb of medium shrimp, without veins or shells
- ½ tsp of salt
- 1 tsp of black pepper
- 1 ½ tsp of paprika
- ½ tsp of garlic powder
- ½ tsp of onion powder
- Cooking spray
- Storage bag

Directions

1. Put the shrimp in the storage bag, and add the ingredients.

2. Seal the bag and shake until the shrimp is covered with the ingredients. Place in the fridge for a half hour.

3. Then, spray the grill and preheat on high. Put shrimp into the grill and cook for about five minutes, or until firm and opaque. Serve and enjoy.

Chickpea and Avocado Panini

This panini is a delicious sandwich for vegetarians and meat eaters alike, because it packs plenty of flavor.

What You Need for the Avocado and Chickpeas

- 15 oz of chickpeas, drained, peeled, and rinsed
- 1 large avocado, peeled, pitted, and quartered
- 2 tbsp of basil, chopped
- 2 tbsp of Italian parsley, chopped
- 2 tbsp of chopped scallions
- 2 tbsp of lemon juice
- Salt and black pepper to taste

What You Need for Panini

- 4 tbsp of room temperature butter
- 8 slices of Italian bread.
- 4 tbsp of basil pesto
- ¼ cup of roasted red bell peppers, sliced
- 4 oz of sliced sharp cheese, such as Asiago
- 4 tablespoons basil pesto
- 1/4 cup sliced roasted red bell peppers
- 4 ounces Asiago or other sharp cheese, sliced

Directions

1. Heat your panini press to a medium-high.

2. While it's heating, mash your chickpeas and avocado together. It can be chunky.

3. Add in the parsley, basil, scallions, and lemon juice, seasoning with salt and pepper.

4. Spread your butter on the bread slices. Then, flip them over and spread pesto on the other side.

5. Add cheese to one slice as well as the smashed chickpeas and avocados, bell peppers, and even more cheese. Close your sandwich with the other side, making sure the buttered side faces up.

6. Put them in the press with the lid closed. Grill for about five minutes, or until the bread is toasted and your cheese is melted.

Sweet Pork Chops

These pork chops are not only delicious, but can be cooked on your presser.

What You Need

- 2 center cut pork chops, around 4 oz a piece.
- ¼ cup of brown sugar
- 2 tbsp of vegetable oil
- 1 tbsp of soy sauce
- 1 tsp of honey
- 1 tbsp of cornstarch
- ¼ cup of water
- A pinch of salt and black pepper

Directions

1. Mix your vegetable oil, sugar, honey, soy sauce, and salt and pepper in a saucepan, and then bring it to a boil.

2. In another cup, mix water and cornstarch.

3. Slowly pour your well-whisked mixture into the saucepan. Set it aside.

4. Meanwhile, preheat your grill on medium-high.

5. Put the pork chops on the press, and close the lid. Grill it for about 8 minutes, and then open up the lid.

6. Brush your pork chops with your mixture. Cook for a couple more minutes, making sure that your mixture doesn't born.

7. When done, remove them from the grill and pour the mix on it.

Classy Steak

Now you don't have to go to an expensive steakhouse to get some steaks. You can make a quality cut from home, and it'll be on the same level as a $30 steak you get at a steakhouse.

What You Need

- 1 8 oz sirloin

- Some olive oil

- 1 clove of garlic

- Salt and black pepper

Directions

1. Preheat grill on medium high. While it's heating, pound your steak with a meat hammer.

2. Make sure it's about ½ inch thick. Cut six slits on each side, and fill it with garlic.

3. Use your brush and cover both sides with olive oil. Make sure you season it with some salt and pepper.

4. Put the steak in the grill. For a medium-rare steak, do it for 4-7 minutes.

5. Do it from 6-9 for medium, or more if you like yours fully cooked. Let steak cool for five minutes before you serve.

Honey and Ginger Salmon

Gotta love some delicious salmon, right? This recipe is lean and good for you. For best results, use smaller pieces so that it's easier to grill.

What You Need

- 2 fillets of salmon
- 2 tbsp of soy sauce
- 1 tsp of garlic powder
- 3 tbsp of honey
- ½ tsp of ground ginger
- ¼ cup of orange juice
- 1 green onion, chopped

Directions

1. Combine soy sauce, garlic, honey, ginger, orange juice, and onion, all in a baking dish.

2. Take out a cup to use later. Put in your fillets and marinate for about 30 minutes.

3. After it's getting close, preheat your grill on high.

4. Add your fillets and close the lid.

5. Grill for about 5-8 minutes.

6. To figure out when it's done, use your fork and see if it flakes. If it flakes with ease, it's done.

7. Put on the rest of your marinade when it's the last minute of your grilling. Serve.

Chapter 5 – Dessert!

If you believe that your press can only make meals and not dessert, you couldn't be more wrong. With a panini press or indoor grill, you can make so many delicious desserts that it will satisfy anyone's sweet tooth. From chocolate to even cakes, there's something in here for everyone.

Dessert is seen by many to be a reward. You shouldn't eat a sweet treat every day, after all. But when you have a craving, it can't be helped. This chapter will cover some that you can make, and even some healthier options involving fruit.

Nutella Chocolate Death Panini

You heard that right. Everyone's favorite spread has its own panini, and it is tasty!

What You Need:

- 8 slices of enriched bread, i.e. challah or brioche
- 8 tbsp of Nutella. Substitute another chocolate spread if you don't want Nutella
- 4 tbsp of small chocolate chips

Directions

1. Preheat your press to high.

2. While it's heating, grab two slices of bread and spread your Nutella on each of them, a tablespoon apiece.

3. Pour a tbsp. of chocolate chips and close the slices.

4. Put two slices in there at a time.

5. Close the lid. It should take about a minute.

6. Don't grill it for an excessive amount of time, or your chocolate chips could melt.

Grilled Peach Delight

Yes, you can even grill fruit on a press. This is ideal if you want a healthy dessert.

What You Need

- 6 firm and ripe large peaches
- 12 oz of fresh or frozen raspberries
- 3 tbsp water
- 1 ½ tbsp. sugar
- 8 oz of mascarpone cheese
- ¾ cup of heavy cream

- ¼ cup of sugar to taste
- 1 tsp vanilla extract

Directions

1. Preheat your grill to medium.

2. Meanwhile, cut your peaches in half, starting at top.

3. Remove the pits, and cut each half into fourths.

4. Put the peaches in the grill on their sides on the grates.

5. Grill for 3-5 minutes until they have grill marks and are tender.

6. Make sure to grill the other side.

7. Meanwhile, make a puree of sugar, water, and raspberries until it's smooth. Strain through a mesh strainer so that the seeds are gone. Press your solids so that you get lots of sauce. This sauce can be refrigerated for two days.

8. To make the whip, combine cream, vanilla, ¼ cup of sugar, and mascarpone.

9. Beat it with an electric mixer until you see firm peaks. You can refrigerate this mixture for two hours.

10. Serve a dollop with grilled peaches and a drizzle of sauce.

For the mascarpone whip:

1. In a medium bowl, combine the mascarpone, heavy cream, vanilla, and remaining 1/4 cup of sugar.

2. Beat the mascarpone mixture with an electric mixer until medium-firm peaks form. This can be made ahead and refrigerated for a few hours.

Ice Cream Cones

Yes, you can make your own ice cream cones in your press! These are delicious and beat the store-bought kind.

What You Need

- 1 cup of heavy cream
- 1 ½ tsp vanilla extract
- 1 ½ cups of powdered sugar
- 1 ½ cups of all-purpose flower
- ¼ tsp of ground cinnamon
- A pinch of ground nutmeg

- 1 tbsp of ground cornstarch
- Wax paper
- Cone mold

Directions

1. Whip your cream and vanilla until it forms a mousse.

2. In another bowl, sift your dry ingredients. Then, add them to the cream and stir until you form a batter.

3. Allow the batter to sit for a half hour.

4. Once it's close to 30 minutes, preheat your grill to medium high.

5. Add a big tablespoon of your batter onto the grill and close your lid, pressing it down.

6. Grill for a minute and a half until it's browned but still can be bent into a shape.

7. Put the pressed cone onto a piece of waxed paper.

8. Using a cone mold, position it in the center of the cone.

9. Roll your cone around the cone mold, making sure that you do it carefully, as it may be hot.

10. Leave it there for ten seconds so that it stays in shape.

11. Repeat with the rest of the batter. Put some ice cream in it and enjoy!

Donut Chips

These make a quick snack to munch on, and they're delicious.

What You Need

- 25 soft glazed donut holes.
- ¼ cup of cinnamon sugar

Directions

1. Preheat your press to medium.

2. Meanwhile, cut each hole in half and cover both sides with cinnamon sugar.

3. Put the halves cut side up on the press, in batches.

4. Close and toast for about 40 seconds.

5. Once that happens, transfer chips onto rack so they can cool. Once they're cool, enjoy.

Mini Yellow Layer Cake with Chocolate Buttercream

We've saved the best for last. This cake is small, but packs a punch. It's great for a party or serving a quick treat for anyone's sweet tooth.

What You Need for the Cake

- 1 egg
- 2 tbsp of sugar
- 2 tbsp of melted butter
- 1 tsp of vanilla extract
- ¼ cup of all-purpose flower
- ¼ big teaspoon of baking powder
- A pinch of salt
- 1 ½ tbsp. of milk

What You Need for the Buttercream

- 3 tbsp of melted unsalted butter
- 3 tbsp of cocoa

- 1 cup powdered sugar, sifted

- 1 ½ tbsp. of milk

- ¼ tsp of vanilla extract

Directions for Yellow Cake

1. Preheat the panini grill at about 350 F.

2. Make sure your grill is flat and not tilted.

3. Spray two 6 oz ramekins with baking spray.

4. Then, in a small bowl, combine the egg and sugar with a whisk.

5. Add vanilla and butter, then mix in your baking powder, flour, and salt.

6. When the batter is smooth, add the milk.

7. Divide your batter in equal parts in the ramekins, about halfway.

8. Lay your ramekins on the grill and close your lid. The upper grates should contact the ramekins' upper edges. Bake for about 17-19 minutes, or until the cake spring back when touched. Let them cool for five minutes in the ramekins and then put them on a rack and let them cool some more.

Directions on Buttercream

1. Combine butter and cocoa.

2. Then, add in the powdered sugar, vanilla, and milk, and whisk until smooth.

3. Assemble the layers and frost with chocolate buttercream. Sprinkles are optional, but sure are fun.

4. To make the chocolate buttercream:

5. In a small bowl, whisk together the butter and cocoa. Add in the powdered sugar, milk and vanilla and whisk until the frosting is smooth.

Conclusion

Now you know just how much variety you can cook when you use your grill. You can fry up some crispy bacon, make a killer burrito, grill some shrimp, and even bake your own personal cake. Indoor grilling can be inexpensive, fun, and can save you a night out in the town. If you want to learn more recipes, do your research, or ask a few friends for suggestions. There are hundreds more recipes you can make with your panini press, and this book is just a starter.

Thank you for downloading this book! If you want to learn about all the other books we have to offer, check out our Amazon page. While you're at it, leave a review and tell us what you think. Feedback is important, and gives us more suggestions when writing our next book. Whether it's positive or negative, we'll appreciate honesty.

Now that you know more about indoor grilling, the next step is to try out some of the recipes. Go out and give it your all. Cooking is something that you can get better at, so practice with these recipes, and soon you'll be the family chef who everyone loves. You don't have to have a huge backyard and a bulky grill to make delicious foods. Anyone can make these. A college kid, a person living in the apartment, and even grandpa. It's something that's easy and fun for almost everyone in your family.

Made in the USA
Middletown, DE
14 October 2022